Perception, Practice, Awareness and Acceptance of Patient's Towards Replacement of Missing Teeth and Prosthetic Options

Perception, Practice, Awareness and Acceptance of Patient's Towards Replacement of Missing Teeth and Prosthetic Options

Anupama Aradya
Raghavendra Swamy K. N.
Narahari Ranganatha
Shwetha E.
Koduru Sravani

ELIVA PRESS

ISBN: 978-99949-8-432-9

Cover Design: Eliva Press
Cover Image: Ingimage
Email: info@elivapress.com
Website: www.elivapress.com

This Eliva Press imprint is published by the registered company Eliva Press Global Ltd. part of Eliva Press S.R.L. Publishing Group

The registered company address is: Pope Hennessy Street Level 2, Hennessy Tower Port Louis, Mauritius
Eliva Press S.R.L. Publishing Group address is: Bulevardul Moscova 21, Chisinau, Moldova, Europe

Title- A Hospital based study to evaluate Perception, Practice, Awareness and Acceptance of patients towards replacement of missing teeth and prosthetic options.

Corresponding Author

Dr Anupama Aradya M D S

Assistant professor

Department of Prosthodontics

JSS Dental college and Hospital, A Constituent college of JSS Academy of Higher Education & Research

Mysuru, Karnataka

India -570015

Email- dranupamavenu@gmail.com

Authors

1.Dr Anupama Aradya M D S

Assistant professor

Department of Prosthodontics

JSS Dental college and Hospital, A Constituent college of JSS Academy of Higher Education & Research

Mysuru, Karnataka

India -570015

Email- dranupamavenu@gmail.com

2.Dr.Raghavendra Swamy K N MDS

Professor and Head of the Department

Department of Prosthodontics

JSS Dental college and Hospital,A Constituent college of JSS Academy of Higher Education & Research

Mysuru, Karnataka

India-570015

3.Dr Narahari Ranganatha

Reader

Department of Oral and Maxillofacial Surgery,

Shree Rajarajeswari Dental College and Hospital, Banglore

4.Dr Shwetha E

Senior Lecturer

Department of Periodontology

Sharavathi Dental College and Hospital

Alkola, T H road

Shimoga-577205

5. Dr Koduru Sravani

Lecturer

Department of Periodontics,

Dayananda Sagar College of Dental Sciences (DSCDS), Bengaluru, Karnataka, India

A Hospital based study to evaluate Perception, Practice, Awareness and Acceptance of patients towards replacement of missing teeth and prosthetic options.

Table of Contents **Page Number**

1. Abstract 2
2. Keywords 3
3. Introduction 3
4. Materials and Methods 6
   - Study Population
   - Questionnaire
   - Clinical Examination
5. Results 7
   - Past dental experience
   - Awareness on the dentures
   - Choice of Prostheses
   - Knowledge on regular check-up
   - Prostheses maintenance
   - Source of Information
   - Reasons for not replaced missing teeth
   - Acceptance of the treatment proposed by Prosthodontist
6. Discussion 10
   - Income and Educational level influence on the choice of prostheses
   - Role of oral health schemes
   - Recommendations
   - Role of Health insurances and Dental Camps
7. Future studies 17
8. Limitations 17
9. Conclusion 18
10. References 19
11. Tables 23
12. Figures 30

Abstract

Purpose - The purpose of this study was to evaluate the level of perception, practice, and awareness of population aged 16-84 years toward the presence of missing teeth and prosthodontics treatment options available for replacing those missing teeth . Additionally to evaluate the acceptance level of prosthodontic treatment proposed by prosthodontist during treatment paln.

Study selection- A pre structured multiple choice questionnaire consisting of socio demographic questions were given to random 300 patients after obtaining their informed consent. The questions included in the survey helped to assess the level of knowledge and awareness of patients towards prosthodontic treatment as a whole. Acceptance level of patients for prosthodontic treatment.

Results- All the age group population were aware of missing teeth in their mouth and they are aware of the replacement of those missing teeth also. Among subjects with degree education 18% choice was removable, 38.5% choice was fixed partial denture and other 38.5 % choice was implant option. For 61.6% of the elder group, 47.6% of the middle age group and 32.7% of the younger adults, friends and relatives were the source of information. 79.3% of the total 300 respondents did not accepted proposed treatment plan, while only 20.7% accepted the treatment plan proposed by prosthodontist..

Conclusion- Within the limitations of this study it can be concluded that, an improvement of practice, knowledge and awareness of patients about the prosthodontics treatment has been observed. With respect to the choice of prosthodontics treatment options, elderly age group choice for the treatment options were removable denture. Individuals with higher education selected the fixed denture and the implant as treatment option. Despite the fact that majority of participants in this research study had a positive attitude or reaction towards dental treatment, it is fundamental to understand the reasons for doubts in patients mind with respect to treatment plan acceptance.

Keywords- Knowledge, Prostheses, Attitude, Acceptance, Awareness, Education, Dental health,Prosthesis

INTRODUCTION

The World Health Organization (WHO) defines health as "a state of complete physical, mental and social well-being, not merely the absence of disease or infirmity" (WHO, 1980). Oral health benefits from this contemporary approach to health as well. The psychological makeup of the patient and how it relates to dental health care are recognised in the modern understanding of dentistry.[1]

Health is multifaceted and influenced by a variety of variables, including genetics, lifestyle, environment, socioeconomic level, and others.[2] Maintaining good oral health enables people to maintain their social roles by maintaining a comfortable and functional dentition. [3] It is believed that oral health education is a necessary precursor for health-related behaviour.[4] Awareness is the characteristic or state of knowing something.

Our interactions with others are influenced by our appearance because we live in a social environment.Teeth are crucial for maintaining of a positive self-image. [5,6] The loss of a tooth is an extremely stressful and upsetting occurrence in life that necessitates extensive social and psychological adaptation.[7,8] It has been proposed that people's attitudes regarding dentures and their negative reactions to edentulousness are crucial for determining whether or not they will accept new dentures.[9]

Recently, demands like aesthetics and practical comfort have been elevated in importance and made easier to meet.[10-11] A number of reasons, including poor general health, decreased income, and an accumulation of oral issues, may limit access to dental care. The patient's need for treatment and the patients' objective oral health are two techniques for evaluating treatments for patients other than clinical dental examination by an expert.[12]

Prosthodontics involves the replacement of teeth loss partial or complete edentulous arch and associated structures, in order to restore back function, aesthetic of the patient in the form of removable or fixed Prosthetics.[13,14]

For a specific clinical condition, several prosthetic treatment alternatives might be available, like removable, fixed tooth/teeth or implant-supported prosthesis. Commonly, inception of prosthodontics treatment options have been perceived as an aspect of the specialist's responsibility. In contemporary clinical practice, patients are consecutively speculating a key role in choosing their actual treatment requirements by revealing their predictions and constraints. [15] The three major areas like patient comfort, function, and aesthetics will influence the adequacy of treatment. Patient comfort and function is determined by mechanical and biological components. However, acceptance of the aesthetic aspectof prosthodontics treatment modality is decided by a variety of social, cultural impacts, attitudes and faith of the patient.[16]Patients' attitude in regard to treatment, sustained by means of a questionnaire before the patients receive the treatment, could be a prospective tool to effect satisfaction with the definitive treatment.[17]For an individual to have dental prosthetic treatment, it is expected to have a close correlation with socio-demographic factors such as age, gender, education, financial status, individual interest and their health assurance, and surrounding environment.[15]Knowledge of patients with respect to prosthodontics treatment may have a key role in their prostheses acceptance.[18]

Now a days, from the point of view of occlusion support, adjacent teeth preservation, and avoidance of a removable partial denture the implant supported prostheses can be reviewed as the treatment of choice (RPD).[19-21]

As we know dental implants are connected with improved denture retention, stability, functional efficiency and quality of life.[22]The studies have reported that dental implants for prosthetic rehabilitation is becoming the most preferred choice amongst the patients.[22]In many developing countries, usage of dental implants in restoring missing tooth/teeth is increasing.[22]However, between individuals and countries, the thoughts and knowledge of patients about dental implants varies.[22]In a survey it was found that, only 23.24% of non-rural population heard about dental implant in an Indian study.[23]In another Indian study, it was shown that, only 33% of the participants had heard of dental implants as a treatment modality.[24]It is essential to evaluate patient awareness and knowledge of implant on a regular basis.[25]

The results of this study will aid in determining the degree of awareness, attitudes, and demand regarding prosthodontic treatment options in patients who are partially and entirely edentulous, since the number of available options in both the government and private sectors has expanded nationwide. We also tried to determine whether there is a distinction between the necessity (from the clinician's perspective) and the demand (from the patient's perspective). Additionally, it was anticipated that this would aid in preventing both undertreatment and overtreatment of a particular patient.

Therefore, the present was planned to evaluate the level of practice, knowledge, awareness and acceptance of population aged between 16-84 years, toward the presence of missing teeth and prosthodontics treatment options available for replacing those missing teeth and the factors which prevented them delaying the treatment if any, before they visited the institution for getting done the treatment. Additionally to assess their acceptance level in regards to the prosthodontics treatment plan proposed by prosthodontist.

MATERIALS AND METHODS

Study Population

A cross-sectional epidemiological survey was planned and conducted in a dental college. The questionnaire survey was conducted on the patients who visited the department of Prosthodontics for restoration of missing tooth/teeth.Ethical clearance was obtained from the institution(No-JSS/DCH/Ethical/06/2016-17(2))and with the consent of the patients, this present questionnaire survey was carried out.

Inclusion criteria

1. Patients referred from other department for prosthodontics treatment were included
2. All patients above the age of 18 years visiting the outpatient department of Prosthodontics, who wanted to get their missing tooth/teeth restored, where included.
3. Those patients, who had a previous history of prosthesis and patients who did not had were considered.
4. Patients willing to accept informed consent.

Exclusion criteria

1. Patients who did not agree to answer the questionnaire.

2. Mentally compromised patients

Questionnaire

A pre-structured multiple choice questionnaire consisting of socio demographic questions were given to 300 patients after obtaining their informed consent. The questions included in the survey helped to assess the level of perception, practice, knowledge, awareness and acceptance of patients towards prosthodontic treatment as a whole. Few questions assessed the patients past dental experience, their expectations, knowledge on different prosthesis available and their preferable choice for the treatment available, source of information for the prosthesis and the maintenance requirement of the available prosthesis. Acceptance of the treatment plan proposed by prosthodontist.

<u>Clinical examination</u>

Accordingly age group was classified from young adult (18-35),middle Aged (36-59)elderly (Above 60) and accordingly the education was classified from Illiterate, primary, high school, pre-university and degree. A single trained investigator recorded answers from the patients followed by a clinical examination.

The clinical examination was performed for the studied groups to evaluate the possibilities of prosthetic treatment (RPD, FPD, implant or no clinical need for replacement)

RESULTS

Statistical analysis was carried out for the obtained data by using Statistical Package for Social Sciences software (SPSS version 21.0).

Among 300 participants, 57.30% were male and 42.70% were female **(Fig.1)**. Distribution of patients according to age group, marital status and education **(Fig 2, Fig 3and Fig 4)**

<u>Past dental experience</u>

All the population participated in the study had good past dental experience (T**able 1).**

<u>Awareness on the dentures</u>

Among the illiterate subjects majority of them were aware of the complete denture, remaining 15% illiterate subjects were aware of both complete denture and removable partial denture together, other 15% illiterate were aware of all complete denture , removable partial denture and fixed denture together. 20.9% Subjects of primary and 21.8% subjects of High school education background were aware of both removable and fixed denture. (**Fig.5**)

All the age group population were aware of missing teeth in their mouth and they are aware of the replacement of those missing teeth also. Twelve percent of the total patient were unaware of the replacement of the missing teeth (**Table 2 and Fig. 6).**

Of the total population, 66.3% were aware of complete denture, 49.3% were aware of removable partial denture, 54.3% were aware of the fixed partial denture and 26.3% were aware of the Implants.23% of middle aged and 17.6% of elderly were aware of complete denture, removable partial denture and fixed partial denture together. 20.4% of younger adults were aware of fixed denture and implant together. Whereas, 10.2% of younger and middle aged population were aware of all the available prosthodontics treatment options.(**Table.3**)

Amongst the educated subjects, 14.6% of subjects were aware of both removable and fixed denture together, 12.5% were aware of all removable, fixed and implant together and remaining 13.5% were aware of all the treatment options available20.3% male and 11.7% female group were aware of only complete denture, and 21.1% female and 16.3% male group were aware of both removable and fixed denture. Whereas 10.2% female and 5.8% male group were aware of all the prosthodontics treatment options available.(**Table.4**)

<u>Choice of Prostheses</u>

Among the elder age group, 64.8% subjects choice was removable denture and 20.8% choice was fixed denture, 1.6% choice was implant. 30.6% of the younger adults choice was fixed denture, 57.1% of the younger adults choice was implant. And even most of the middle aged population choice was fixed denture and implant(**Table. 5**)

Among illiterate subjects, 69.7% choice was removable denture, 18.2% choice was fixed denture. Among subjects with primary education 63.7% choice was removable denture, 23.6% choice was fixed partial denture. Among subjects with high school education 36.3% choice was removable denture, 29.7% choice was fixed partial denture, Among subjects with pre university education 32% choice was removable 32 % choice was fixed partial denture and 28% choice was implant. Among subjects with degree education 18% choice was removable, 38.5% choice was fixed partial denture and other 38.5 % choice was implant option.(**Table.6**)

Compare to the male group female group opted for fixed partial denture and implant option for the replacement.(**Table 7**)

Knowledge on regular check-up

Interestingly 81% of the total population believe in regular visit for dental check-up.14.7% individuals wants to visit on requirement. In gender category there was common opinion on the regular visit for check up.

Prostheses Maintenance

Most of the population believe in the maintenance of the prostheses. Both female and male group believe in the maintenance of the prostheses

Source of Information

For 61.6% of the elder group, 47.6% of the middle age group and 32.7% of the younger adults, friends and relatives were the source of information. For 49.0%elder group, 29.4% middle age group and 24.0% younger adults, Dentists were source of information, For 75.8% illiterate subjects and 61.8% subjects with primary education, 53.8% subjects with high school education, 48% with pre university education friends and relatives were source of information. For 45.8% subjects with degree dentists are the source of information. For 53.1% female and 49.4% male group, friends and relatives are the source of information.(**Table.8 and table.9**)

Reasons for not replaced missing teeth

Out of total population, 23.3% gave the reason of financial constraint, 13.3% reason was inadequate knowledge and 12.7% were not motivated. 30.3% of the illiterate subjects were not motivated, 30.2% subjects with degree education gave the reason of financial constraint. 24.2% female and 22.7% male group gave the reason of financial constraint.(**Table. 10**)

Acceptance of the treatment proposed by Prosthodontist

From among the 300 participants, 172 were males and 128 were females. 79% of the total 300 respondents did not acknowledge or accepted substitute treatment, while only 21% accepted the treatment plan suggested by the dental specialist. (**Fig.9**)

DISCUSSION

In a highly populated country like India, statistical analysis on patients' practice, knowledge, awareness, and acceptance towards tooth replacement is minimal. So, an attempt was made to find out the level of practice, knowledge, awareness and acceptance towards the replacement of teeth among patients.

Since the patients in our study had reported on their own to the hospital for replacement of teeth, it was expected to find that all the subjects expressed their missing teeth had to be replaced, but 12% of the population was unaware of replacement of teeth because they had no missing teeth so the higher level of awareness in these populations is required during routine dental consultations and educative counselling during these consultations.

The study done ten years back on prosthodontic awareness has shown that there was lack of awareness about prosthodontic treatment but in comparison to previous study,the present study has shown a increase in the awareness amongst the individuals.[26]So compare to ten years back study, there is a positive impact on the knowledge of Prosthodontic restoration status.(**Table.2**)

While the removable prosthodontics options were known to most of the patients(66.3%), their awareness on fixed partial denture(54.3%), tooth and implant supported prostheses (26.3%), was also at a higher level(**Fig.6**).Younger and middle aged population((10.2%) were aware of all the prosthodontics treatment options available. Similar findings were observed in a study conducted by Suprakash *et al.,* (2013), age also showed differences in treatment wise as younger people being more enthusiastic and educated were having knowledge for this treatment in large numbers. [25]

Compare to ten years back study done by Chowdhary et al, [24]our study results have shown that younger adults are aware of implant supported prostheses there is a percentage of growth in awareness of implant restoration among the individuals, but their study was on multicenters. Future study has to be conducted for the same at various multicenters

Similar toNomura et al,[19] study our study has shown that the likelihood of attending prosthodontics treatment is related to sociodemographic background.Education is a key factor in the prosthesis consultation.[27]In their study, Shah *et al.* reported that the prevalence of wearing of dentures increased with the increase in the level of literacy.[28] It may be that individuals with higher educational achievements have greater health concerns and thus seek prosthodontics care more often than those with lower levels of education. High level of education may be one of the main reasons that majority of population with education of degree were aware of all the prosthodontics treatment options available.

Both female and male group had the awareness on the missing teeth. In case of knowledge on prosthodontics treatment options available, female had the knowledge on all the treatment options available compare to male group. Female group were aware of both removable and fixed denture available. Similarly females having more knowledge as compared to males, these findings are similar to this study.[29] In another study while 26 females and 17 males were prefer FPD as treatment modalities.[18]

Interestingly all the participants were familiar with the college and hospital where the treatment can be taken.Most of the patients opted to get treated from the dental college than private clinics; this may be to reduce the financial burden following a prosthetic replacement. In the current study majority of the elderly age group choice for the treatment options were removable denture as they were more aware of it, some of the individuals who have already been rehabilitated, the denture is most frequently used and they were comfortable and familiar with the removable denture as it is inexpensive and seems more accessible to them depending on their socio-economical level.[31]Although 20.8% elder individuals choice was fixed denture and similar to other study the implant choice was less in this age group so education and motivation is required for this group regarding implant.[37]Whereas younger age group majority of them opted implant and remaining participants fixed prostheses this may be due to the increase in technology and media.In addition, young people are more concerned about their appearance and teeth.**(Table. 5**)

Even though there is a scarcity of data regarding patient's preferences in field of fixed prosthodontics, this study shows an increase in demand for fixed partial denture by the individual with knowledge of the same.(**Fig.7**)

Income and Educational level influence on the choice of prostheses

Income and educational status of individuals are often correlated. Majority of the Illiterate individuals opted the removable dentures, they may be familiar with the existing dentures or may be the financial constraint to opt for the fixed denture. Individuals with degree education selected the fixed denture and the implant as treatment option, it may be that individuals with higher educational attainments have greater health concerns and thus seek prosthodontics care more often than those with lower levels of education.[28]**(Table 6 and Fig.5**)

We consider the fact that more than 95% of the participants were aware that regular dental visits are required in order to maintain optimum oral and dental health of an individual to be a positive factor. The participants' awareness of regular dental visits was also assessed according to variables such as gender, age and educational level and the results revealed that it is statistically significant when gender, ethnicity and the educational levels were considered.

More than 95% of the individuals believe in the maintenance of the prostheses.

For majority of the individualsfriends and relatives are the source of information. Similar to other study this claim is supported by the fact that most of the patients (about 34%) highlighted that their source of information on prosthodontics options was friends or relatives. [32]Whereas for subjects with degree education, dentists are the source of information because they may be visiting the dentists regularly, so here it is very important for the dentists to educate and motivate the patient during clinical examination itself regarding the awareness, need for prosthodontics treatment, different treatment options available, maintenance of oral hygiene as well as prostheses . However, a study by Mukatash *et al.,*[14] carried out in Jordan found that the major source of information for patients is dentists. Similarly other study highlights the significant role that the dentists play a vital role in the spread of awareness about prosthodontics treatment and they prove a good source of information which facilitates further spread of information to patient's friends and relatives. Like other study, [32] our study reveal that mass media does not play a significant role in the education on prosthodontics aspects of dental health. Hence media can play a role in educating the public about dental treatment options for missing teeth.(**Fig.8**)

In agreement with the findings of other studies, [33,34]the current study shows majority of them gave the reason of financial constraint for not replacing the teeth even though they had the knowledge (**Table.10**). Illiterate individuals were not motivated for replacement of teeth, so here dental health check-up camps play a vital role, as well as the mass media and dentists are very important to motivate them. Health insurances should provide benefits to prosthodontics rehabilitation and other dental treatment as well.

In our investigation just 20.7% agreed to get the prosthodontics treatment done, but, majority of the patients declined proposed treatment plan (79.3%) (**Fig.9**) as a result of various factors not permitting them to acknowledge the treatment.

Youthful individuals opted to get the treatment since people in their twenties generally care much about their appearance and they are additionally extremely dynamic to get the dental treatment in similar to Jung HK et al study. [35] Individuals with degree education opted to get the treatment than the people without the schooling. The current investigation shows that unmarried individuals opted to get more prosthetic treatment than married individuals with statistically significance which is in contrast with Jung HK et al study.[35] Male patients opted to receive the treatment than females which is in contrast with Shrirao, *et al.* study. [36]

Role of Oral Health Schemes

In India, overall coverage of dental health insurance is low; approximately 10 percent of the population is assessed to approach health insurance coverage. Generally, the health care demands of the rural poor individuals and informal workers have been to a great extent neglected. In spite of, several initiatives have been tried. Danta Bhagya yojana an oral health intiative by Karnataka State Government provide free dentures to the senior citizens with complete tooth loss(aged 60 or above) belonging to the below poverty line families. The scheme was launched in 2014 December and is aimed at providing free dentures to at least 30,000 senior citizens. The State Government has involved 45 government and private dental colleges in the State to implement the Danta Bhagya scheme. Our Institution is one among them to rehabilitate the individuals under Danta Bhagya Yojana. The scheme provided free denture to patient above 60 years of age and residing in Karnataka with BPL card holder. Modification was done with regarding the age group and reduced to 45 years so as to provide free denture to a larger population and partial denture was also included in the scheme for loss of more than 3 teeth. This oral health policy will have a positive impact on the state of dental health in the State.

Recommendations

Here are a few recommendations to accept the treatment and to improve their oral health status. Initially, it is necessary for those who are older and less educated to provide oral health education,and importance of dental prosthetic treatment because they demand more prosthetic treatment. Second, for those who need prosthetic treatment but cannot afford the treatment, government intervention, such as enacting an oral health initiative for alienated group's prosthetic treatments is necessary. Third, dental professionals and people related to dental field have responsibilities to inform the public of improvement of chewing by prosthetic treatment. Moreover, dental health insurance should discover a place in the schemes proposed by the government public authority circumstance so that individuals can afford to get the dental treatment which is ideal for them.

Other recommendation is that the Danta Bhagya scheme should broaden their facilities like giving fixed partial denture and systemic community based oral health promotion ought to be reinforced, which stress upon the potential outcomes and constraints of any prosthetic replacement a patient may prefer using distinctive accessible media.

Role of Health Insurance and Dental Camps

Dental schooling camps, utilization of print media like newspapers, promotions, banners, and visual media, for example, short movies and recordings should be done for the same for creating mass awareness of the treatment methods and their advantages during this pandemic circumstance. Economic stressors in general populace will require relief and fast changes in policy would help. Mobile dental vans, giving on-site dental treatment, might be a plausible arrangement.

So systemic community-based oral health promotion should be strengthened, which stress upon the possibilities and limitations of any prosthetic replacement a patient may prefer utilizing different available media.

The majority of patients that visited our prosthodontics out-patient department (OPD) are from the rural areas in and around Mysore. Most of these patients still follow ancient traditions passed down from generations, with more emphasis on general health rather than oral health. Hence formulating a treatment plan that satisfies both the patients expectations and treatment plan laid out by the dentist is difficult.

The decision to become edentulous is influenced by a number of non-disease factors, including attitude, behaviour, dental attendance, and aspects of the healthcare system, according to research. Additionally, there is a significant link between the edentulous state and the financial issues that are typically connected to poor occupational levels. It is fair to infer that edentulism is caused by a variety of confluences of cultural, educational, economical, and dental disease attitude variables, as well as by previous treatment. [37]

Future Studies

Future studies should determine how the dental profession and society might address an increased demand for services among people who have limited financial resources. These studies would provide important insights into the various types of assistance and insurance programs that might be designed and implemented to benefit each individual. Future surveys can be carried out from various demographically different locations. Further studies can be done to know the reasons for not accepting the proposed treatment plan.

Limitations

1. The survey was taken from the patients who visited only one Dental college.
2. Limited sample size and institutional setup where prosthetic treatment charges are less as compared to private dental care centres

3. Reasons for not accepting the treatment plan proposed by prosthodontist was not assessed

CONCLUSION

Within the limitations of this study it can be concluded that,

- Practice, awareness and knowledge of patients and choice of patients regarding prosthodontics treatment are different among age group, gender, education of populations.
- The removable prosthodontics options were known to most of the patients, their awareness on fixed partial denture, and implant supported prostheses , was also at a higher level with respect to the knowledge and awareness of patients about the prosthodontics treatment ,
- elderly age group choice for the treatment options were removable denture as they were more aware of it, as it is inexpensive and seems more accessible to them depending on their socio-economical level but the implant choice was less in this age group so education and motivation is required for this group regarding implant with respect to the choice of prosthodontics treatment options,
- Individuals with higher educational attainments have greater health concerns and thus seek prosthodontics care more often than those with lower levels of education
- Friends and relatives are the most common source of information for the patients in terms of education about different treatment options available to replace the missing teeth.

- Regular dental visits are required in order to maintain optimum oral and dental health of an individual to be a positive factor and the patients believe in maintenance of the prostheses as well.
- Despite the fact that majority of participants in this research study had a positive attitude or reaction towards dental treatment, it is fundamental to understand the reasons for doubts in patients mind with respect to treatment plan acceptance.

References

1. van Waas MA. The influence of psychologic factors on patient satisfaction with complete dentures. J Prosthet Dent 1990;63:545-8.
2. Mahajan BK. Social environment. Textbook of Preventive and Social Medicine. 1st ed. New Delhi: Jaypee Brothers Medical Publishers (P) Ltd.; 1991. p. 82-7.
3. Ashley FP. Role of dental health education in preventive dentistry. In: Murray JJ, editor. Prevention of Dental Disease. 3rd ed. Oxford: Oxford University Press; 1996. p. 406-14.
4. Wright FA. Children's perception of vulnerability to illness and dental
5. disease. Community Dent Oral Epidemiol 1982;10:29-32
6. Levinson NA. Psychological facets of Esthetic dental health care: A developmental perspective. J Prosthet Dent 1990;64:486-91.
7. Roessler DM. Complete denture success for patients and dentists. Int Dent J 2003;53:340-5.
8. Omar R, Tashkandi E, Abduljabbar T, Abdullah MA, Akeel RF. Sentiments expressed in relation to tooth loss: A qualitative study among edentulous Saudis. Int J Prosthodont 2003;16:515-20.
9. Fiske J, Davis DM, Frances C, Gelbier S. The emotional effects of tooth loss in edentulous people. Br Dent J 1998;184:90-3.
10. al Quran F, Clifford T, Cooper C, Lamey PJ. Influence of psychological factors on the acceptance of complete dentures. Gerodontology 2001;18:35-40.

11. Käyser AF. Shortened dental arches and oral function. J Oral Rehabil 1981;8:457-62.
12. Witter DJ, Van Elteren P, Käyser AF, Van Rossun GM. The effect of removable partial dentures on the oral function in shortened dental arches. J Oral Rehabil 1989;16:27-33.
13. Kalk W, Käyser AF, Witter DJ. Needs for tooth replacement. Int Dent J 1993;43:41-9.
14. Carlsson GE. Omar R. Trends in prosthodontics. *Med Princ Pract* 2006; **5(3)**:167-179.
15. Mukatash GN, Al-Rousan M, Al-Sakarna B. Needs and demands of prosthetic treatment among two groups of individuals. *Indian J Dental Res* 2010; **21(4)**:564.
16. Leles CR, Freire Mdo C. A sociodental approach in prosthodontic treatment decision making. *J Appl Oral Sci* 2004;**12**:127-132.
17. Conny DJ, Tedesco LA, Brewer JD, Albino JE. Changes of attitude in fixed prosthodontic patients. *J Prosthet Dent* 1985;**53**:451-454.
18. van Waas MA. Determinants of dissatisfaction with dentures: A multiple regression analysis. *J Prosthet Dent* 1990;**64**:569-572.
19. Shigli K, Angadi GS, Hebbal M. Knowledge of prosthodontics treatment among denture - wearers and non - denture - wearers attending a dental institute in India: a survey report. *Gerodontology* 2007; **24(4)**:211-216.
20. Stanford CM. Application of oral implants to the general dental practice. *J Am Dent Assoc* 2005; **136**:1092-1100.
21. Jivraj S, Chee W. Treatment planning of implants in posterior quadrants. *Br Dent J* 2006;**201**:13-23.
22. Davenport JC, Basker RM, Heath JR, Ralph JP, Glantz PO. Need and demand for treatment. *Br Dent J* 2000;**189**:364 -368.
23. Al-Johany S, Al Zoman HA, Al Juhaini M, Al Refeai M. Dental patients' awareness and knowledge in using dental implants as an option in replacing missing teeth: A survey in Riyadh, Saudi Arabia. *Saudi Dent J*2010; **22**: 183-188.

24. Chowdhary R, Mankani N, Chandraker NK. Awareness of dental implants as a treatment choice in urban Indian populations. *Int J Oral Maxillofac Implants*2010;**25**: 305-308.

25. Suprakash B, Ahammad A, Yusuf R, Amit T, Raghavendra K, et al. Knowledge and attitude of patients toward dental implants as an option for replacement of missing teeth. *J Contemp Dent Pract*2013; **14**: 115-118.

26. Guyatt GH, Cook DJ. Health status, quality of life, and the individual. *JAMA* 1994; **272**: 630-631.

27. Singh SV, Tripathi A. A study on prosthodontic awareness and needs of an aging Indian rural population. J Indian Prosthodont Soc 2007;7(1):21-23.

28. Meriem Amine, Azzaz Amine, Bouhaji M, Sarah Saif, Serrhier Z, Bennani Anas et al., Needs and Demands in Prosthetic Treatment in the Population Followed within the Prosthetic Department of Casablanca's Dental Consultation and Treatment Center. *Int J Dentistry Oral Sci* 2016; **03(2)**: 200-204.

29. Shah N, Parkash H, Sunderam R. Edentulousness, denture wear and denture needs of Indian elderly- a community based study. *J Oral Rehabil*2004; **31**: 467–476.

30. Abdurahiman VT, Abdul Khader M, Sanju John Jolly. Frequency of partial edentulism and awareness to restore the same: a cross sectional study in the age group of 18-25 years among Kerala student population. *J Indian Prosthodont Soc* 2013; **13**: 46-65.

31. Memon F, Khatri DR, Memon S. Prosthodontic treatment; clinical evaluation of the preference for prosthodontic treatment modalities in the patients visiting at the Isra Dental College, Hyderabad. *Professional Med J* 2018; **25(7)**:1034-1040.

32. Hescot P, Bourgeois D, Doury J. Oral health in 35–44-year-old adults in France. *Int Dent J* 1997; **47(2)**: 94-99.

33. Jayasinghe R, Janana Perera, Jayasinghe V, Thilakumara I, Rasnayaka S, ShirazMHM, et al. Awareness, attitudes, need and demand on replacement of missing teeth among a group of partially dentate patients attending a University Dental Hospital.*BMC Res Notes* 2017; **10**:334
34. Raj N, Reddy N, Japatti S, Thomas M, Uthappa R. Knowledge, attitudes towards prosthodontics rehabilitation and utilization of dental services among Songadh and Amargadh Population. *J Dent Med Med Sci* 2014;3(1):1–6.
35. Shigli K, Hebbal M, Angadi GS. Attitudes towards replacement of teeth among patients at the Institute of Dental Sciences, Belgaum, India.*J Dent Educ*2007 ;**71(11):**1467-1475.
36. Jung HK, Kim HG. Factors affecting patients decision-making for dental Prosthetic treatment. *J Korean Acad Prosthodont* 2008;46:610-20.
37. Shrirao ND, Deshmukh SP, Pande NA, Radke UM. An evaluation of patient's decisions regarding dental prosthetic treatment. *JIndian Prosthodont Soc* 2016;16:366-71.

Source of fund: (if any): Nil

Conflict of interest: The authors declare that there is no conflicts of interests among them.

Ethical clearance: The study participant (Patient)was informed and a written informed consent fortheir willingness to publish the data was obtained.

Tables

		Count	Percentage %
Past Dental Experience	Bad	3	1.0%
	Good	182	60.7%
	Nil	27	9.0%
	Satisfactory	45	15.0%
	Very Good	43	14.3%

Table 1- Past dental experience of the participants

		Count	Percentage %
Are you aware that missing teeth have to be replaced	Yes	264	88.0%
	No	36	12.0%

Table 2- Awareness of missing teeth

		Age					
		Young adult(18-35)		Middle Aged (36-59)		Elderly (Above 60)	
		N	%	N	%	N	%
Awareness on available prostheses	a	1	2.0%	15	11.9%	34	27.4%
	b	1	2.0%	4	3.2%	1	0.8%
	c	2	4.1%	4	3.2%	3	2.4%
	d	3	6.1%	0	0.0%	2	1.6%
	e	4	8.2%	18	14.3%	16	12.8%
	a,b	0	0.0%	11	8.7%	23	19.2%
	a,c	3	6.0%	3	2.4%	8	6.4%
	a,d	0	0.0%	1	0.8%	0	0.0%
	b,c	3	6.0%	6	4.8%	5	4.0%
	c,d	10	20.4%	5	4.0%	1	0.8%
	a,b,c	3	6.0%	29	23.0%	22	17.6%
	a,b,d	0	0.0%	1	0.8%	1	0.8%
	a,b,c	0	0.0%	0	0.0%	1	0.8%
	a,c,d	7	14.3%	10	7.9%	2	1.6%
	b,c,d	7	14.3%	6	4.8%	0	0.0%
	a,b,c,d	5	10.2%	13	10.3%	5	4.0%

Table 3- Awareness of different age group population on available prostheses (a. Complete Denture, b. Removable Partial Denture, c. Fixed Partial Denture, d. Implant e. Not aware)

		Education									
		Degree		High School		Illiterate		Pre University		Primary	
		N	%	N	%	N	%	N	%	N	%
Awareness on available prostheses	a	9	9.4%	13	14.3%	14	42.4%	4	16.0%	10	18.2%
	b	0	0.0%	1	1.1%	2	6.1%	1	4.0%	2	3.6%
	c	5	5.2%	3	3.3%	0	0.0%	0	0.0%	1	1.8%
	d	2	2.1%	0	0.0%	1	3.0%	1	4.0%	1	1.8%
	e	2	2.1%	24	26.4%	3	9.1%	2	8.0%	7	12.7%
	a,b	2	2.1%	12	13.2%	5	15.2%	3	12.0%	13	23.6%
	a,c	4	4.1%	4	4.4%	0	0.0%	2	8.0%	4	7.3%
	a,d	0	0.0%	1	1.1%	0	0.0%	0	0.0%	0	0.0%
	b,c	8	8.2%	2	2.2%	0	0.0%	2	8.0%	2	3.6%
	c,d	14	14.5%	0	0.0%	1	3.0%	1	4.0%	0	0.0%
	a,b,c	14	14.6%	19	20.9%	5	15.2%	4	16.0%	12	21.8%
	a,b,d	2	2.1%	0	0.0%	0	0.0%	0	0.0%	0	0.0%
	a,c,d	12	12.5%	4	4.4%	1	3.0%	1	4.0%	1	1.8%
	b,c,d	9	9.4%	2	2.2%	0	0.0%	2	8.0%	0	0.0%
	a,b,c	0	0.0%	1	1.1%	0	0.0%	0	0.0%	0	0.0%
	a,b,c,d	13	13.5%	5	5.5%	1	3.0%	2	8.0%	2	3.6%

Table 4- Individuals of different education backround Awareness on available prostheses (a. Complete Denture, b. Removable Partial Denture, c. Fixed Partial Denture, d. Implants e. Not aware)

		Age					
		Young adult(18-35)		Middle Aged (36-59)		Elderly (Above 60)	
		N	%	N	%	N	%
Choice of prostheses	a	0	0.0%	15	11.9%	73	58.4%
	b	1	2.0%	20	15.9%	8	6.4%
	c	15	30.6%	50	39.7%	26	20.8%
	d	28	57.1%	26	20.6%	2	1.6%
	e	4	8.2%	15	11.9%	16	12.8%
	c,d	1	2.0%	0	0.0%	0	0.0%

Chi Square = 73.2 p= 0.0001

Table 5- Individuals of different age group choice of prostheses. (a. Complete Denture, b. Removable Partial Denture, c. Fixed Partial Denture, d. Implants e. No need for repacement)

		education									
		Illiterate		Primary		High School		Pre University		Degree	
		N	%	N	%	N	%	N	%	N	%
Choice of prostheses	a	17	51.5%	26	47.3%	27	29.7%	4	16.0%	14	14.6%
	b	6	18.2%	9	16.4%	6	6.6%	4	16.0%	4	4.2%
	c	6	18.2%	13	23.6%	27	29.7%	8	32.0%	37	38.5%
	d	2	6.1%	1	1.8%	9	9.9%	7	28.0%	37	38.5%
	e	2	6.1%	6	10.9%	21	23.1%	2	8.0%	4	4.2%
	c, d	0	0.0%	0	0.0%	1	1.1%	0	0.0%	0	0.0%

Chi Square = 85.6 p= 0.001

Table 6- Individuals with different education background choice of prostheses. (a. Complete Denture, b. Removable Partial Denture, c. Fixed Partial Denture, d. Implants e. No need for repacement)

		Gender			
		Female		male	
		Count	Percentage %	Count	Percentage%
Choice of prostheses	a	26	20.3%	62	36.0%
	b	14	10.9%	15	8.7%
	c	43	33.6%	48	27.9%
	d	30	23.4%	26	15.1%
	e	14	10.9%	21	12.2%
	c,d	1	0.8%	0	0.0%

Chi Square = 10.1 p= 0.039

Table 7- choice of prostheses in relation to Gender(a. Complete Denture, b. Removable Partial Denture, c. Fixed Partial Denture, d. Implants e. No need for repacement)

		Age					
		Young adult(18-35)		Middle Aged (36-59)		Elderly (Above 60)	
		N	%	N	%	N	%
Source of information	a	0	0.0%	6	4.8%	5	4.0%
	b	4	8.2%	8	6.3%	4	3.2%
	c	3	6.1%	10	7.9%	3	2.4%
	d	24	49.0%	37	29.4%	30	24.0%
	e	16	32.7%	60	47.6%	77	61.6%
	f-doctor	0	0.0%	0	0.0%	2	1.6%
	f-govt hosp	0	0.0%	2	1.6%	0	0.0%
	f-internet	1	2.0%	0	0.0%	0	0.0%
	f-taken treatment for caries	0	0.0%	2	1.6%	1	0.8%
	b,c	1	2.0%	0	0.0%	0	0.0%
	d,e	0	0.0%	1	0.8%	1	0.8%
	d,e	0	0.0%	0	0.0%	1	0.8%
	a.e	0	0.0%	0	0.0%	1	0.8%

Chi Square = 21.7 p=0.017

Table 8- source of information for the available prosthetic options in relation to age(a. Magazines, b.newspapers, c.T.V. and radio, d. Dentist, e. Friends and relatives, f. Other sources)

		Education									
		Degree		High School		Illiterate		Pre University		Primary	
		N	%	N	%	N	%	N	%	N	%
Source of information	a	6	6.2%	2	2.2%	1	3.0%	0	0.0%	2	3.6%
	b	4	4.2%	4	4.4%	2	6.1%	2	8.0%	4	7.3%
	c	4	4.2%	8	8.8%	0	0.0%	2	8.0%	2	3.6%
	d	44	45.8%	24	26.4%	5	15.2%	9	36.0%	9	16.4%
	e	33	34.4%	49	53.8%	25	75.8%	12	48.0%	34	61.8%
	f	0	0.0%	0	0.0%	0	0.0%	0	0.0%	1	1.8%
	f-doctor	1	1.0%	0	0.0%	0	0.0%	0	0.0%	0	0.0%
	f-govt hop	0	0.0%	1	1.1%	0	0.0%	0	0.0%	0	0.0%
	f-govt hosp	0	0.0%	1	1.1%	0	0.0%	0	0.0%	0	0.0%
	f-internet	1	1.0%	0	0.0%	0	0.0%	0	0.0%	0	0.0%
	f-taken treatment for caries	1	1.0%	0	0.0%	0	0.0%	0	0.0%	2	3.6%
	b&c	0	0.0%	1	1.1%	0	0.0%	0	0.0%	0	0.0%
	d,e	1	1.0%	1	1.1%	0	0.0%	0	0.0%	1	1.8%
	a&e	1	1.0%	0	0.0%	0	0.0%	0	0.0%	0	0.0%

Chi Square = 37.8   p= 0.009

Table 9- Individuals with different education group-source of information for the available prostheses. a. Magazines, b.newspapers, c.TV. and radio, d. Dentist, e. Friends and relatives, f. Other sources)

		Count	Percentage %
If you have not replaced Teeth then why	Financial Constraints	70	23.3%
	Inadequate Knowledge	40	13.3%
	Not motivated	38	12.7%
	Other	25	8.2%
	Taking Treatment	127	42.3%

Table 10-Reasons for not replacing the missing teeth among total participants

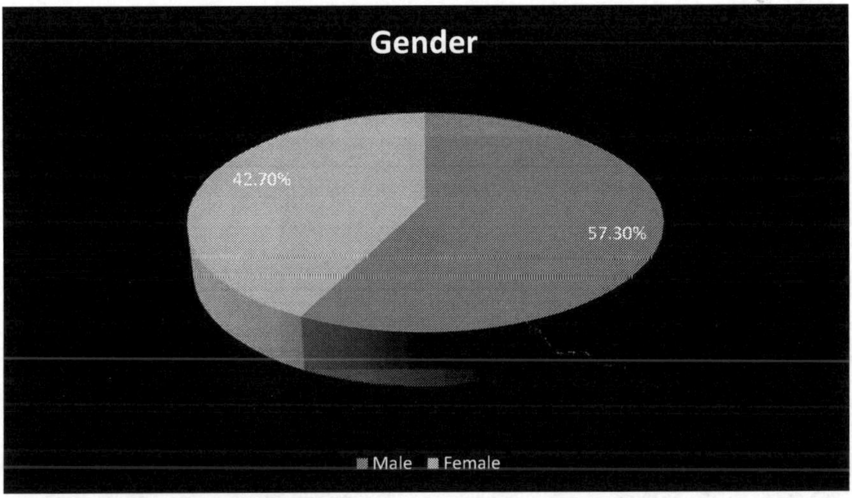

Figure.1- Distribution of patients

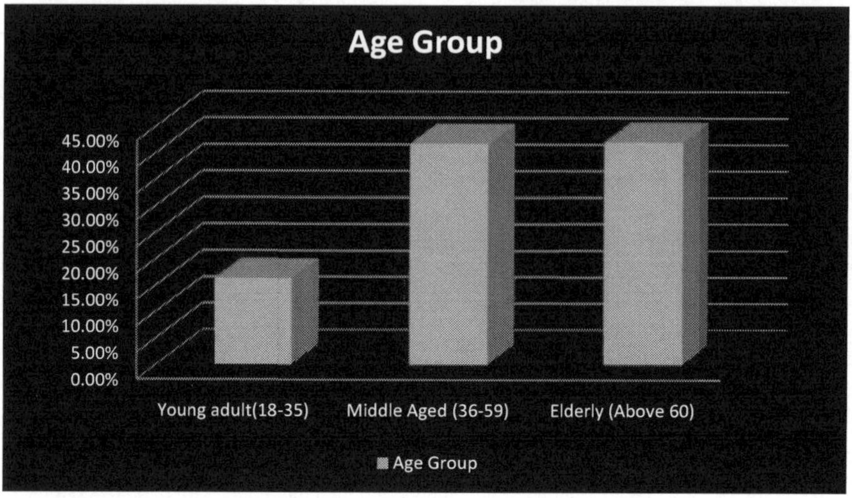

Figure.2- Distribution of patients according to age group

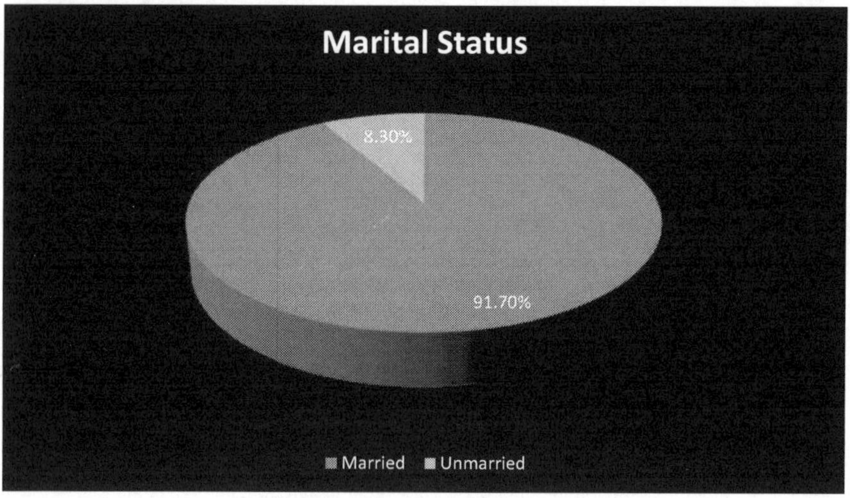

Figure.3- Distribution of individuals on marital status

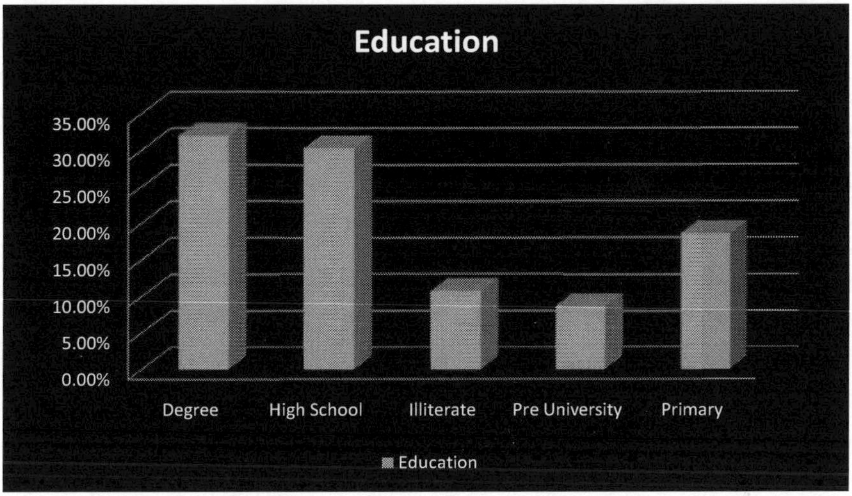

Figure.4- Distribution of patients on education

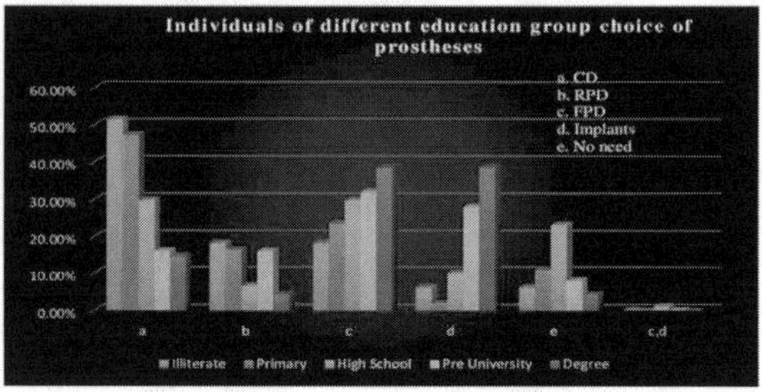

Figure .5-Individuals of different education group of choice of prostheses

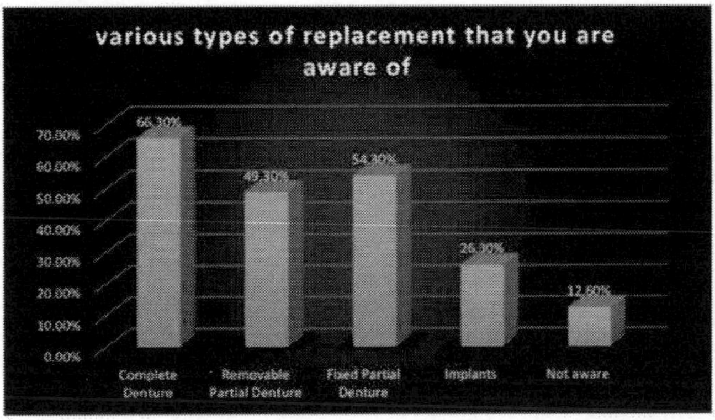

Figure. 6- various types of replacement awareness

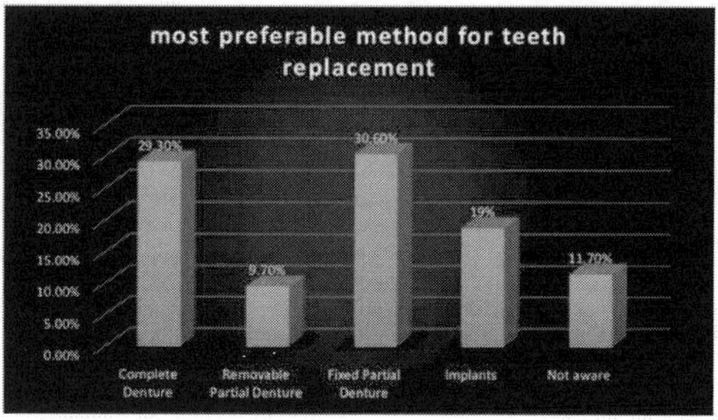

Figure 7-most preferable method for teeth replacement

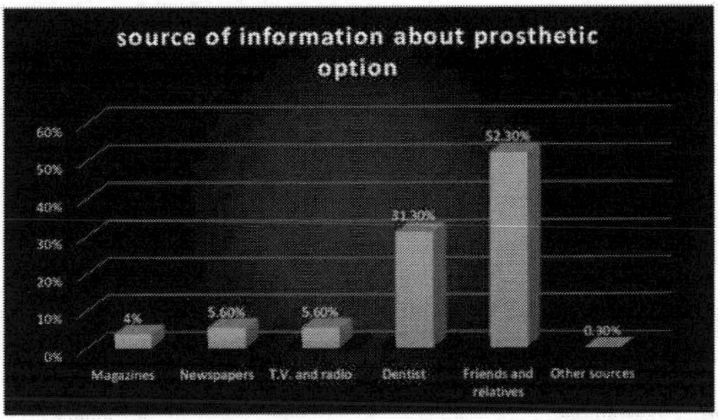

Figure 8-Source of information about prosthetic option

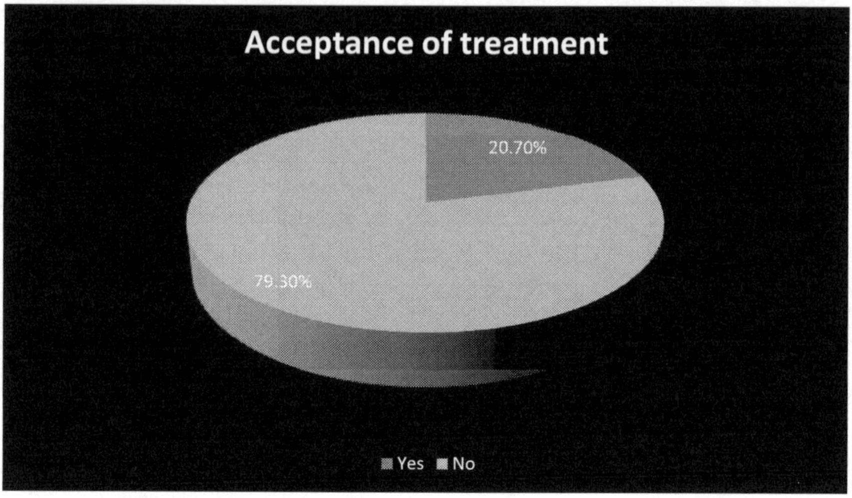

Figure.9- Acceptance of treatment

Legends

Figure.1- Distribution of patients

Figure.2- Distribution of patients according to age group

Figure.3- Distribution of individuals on marital status

Figure.4- Distribution of patients on education

Figure 5-Individuals of different education group of choice of prostheses

Figure 6- various types of replacement awareness

Figure 7-most preferable method for teeth replacement

Figure 8-source of information about prosthetic option

Figure.9- Acceptance of treatment

Tables

Table 1- Past dental experience of the participants

Table 2- Awareness of missing teeth

Table 3- Awareness of different age group population on available prostheses (a. Complete Denture, b. Removable Partial Denture, c. Fixed Partial Denture, d. Implant e. Not aware)

Table 4- Individuals of different education backround Awareness on available prostheses (a. Complete Denture, b. Removable Partial Denture, c. Fixed Partial Denture, d. Implants e. Not aware)

Table 5- Individuals of different age group choice of prostheses. (a. Complete Denture, b. Removable Partial Denture, c. Fixed Partial Denture, d. Implants e. No need for repacement)

Table 6- Individuals with different education background choice of prostheses. (a. Complete Denture, b. Removable Partial Denture, c. Fixed Partial Denture, d. Implants e. No need for repacement)

Table 7- choice of prostheses in relation to Gender(a. Complete Denture, b. Removable Partial Denture, c. Fixed Partial Denture, d. Implants e. No need for repacement)

Table 8- source of information for the available prosthetic options in relation to age(a. Magazines, b.newspapers, c.T.V. and radio, d. Dentist, e. Friends and relatives, f. Other sources)

Table 9- Individuals with different education group-source of information for the available prostheses. a. Magazines, b.newspapers, c.T.V. and radio, d. Dentist, e. Friends and relatives, f. Other sources)

Table 10-Reasons for not replacing the missing teeth among total participants

Publisher: Eliva Press Global Ltd

Email: info@elivapress.com

Made in United States
Orlando, FL
04 November 2026

90209892R00026